Sophia's Jungle Adventure

A Fun and Educational Kids Yoga Story

By Giselle Shardlow
Illustrated by Emily Gedzyk

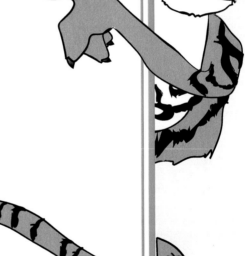

Welcome to..

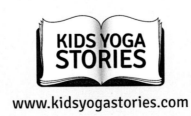

KIDS YOGA STORIES

www.kidsyogastories.com

For my daughter, Anamika, who might one day
become a traveling yogi.

~ G.S. ~

For my mother, who is the most admirable woman I know. And to Dan,
my constant inspiration in life.

~ E.G. ~

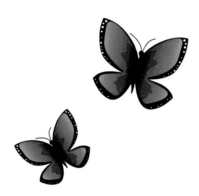

Sophia's Jungle Adventure

Third Edition

Copyright © 2014 by Giselle Shardlow
Cover and illustrations by Emily Gedzyk
All images © 2014 Giselle Shardlow
First published in 2012.

ISBN-13: 978-1475225488
ISBN-10: 1475225482

Kids Yoga Stories
Boston, MA
www.kidsyogastories.com
www.amazon.com/author/giselleshardlow
Email us at info@kidsyogastories.com

Ordering Information: Special discounts are available on quantity purchases by contacting the publisher at the email address above.

What do you think? Let us know what you think of **Sophia's Jungle Adventure** at feedback@kidsyogastories.com.

Printed in the United States of America.

Welcome to a Kids Yoga Stories Book

The **Kids Yoga Stories** series is designed to teach young children to link the interactive movements of yoga to topics of interest while promoting lively, dynamic learning experiences. The stories link several poses in a specific sequence to create a coherent and meaningful story. Each story's objective is to increase comprehension and encourage children's love of reading by actively engaging their minds and bodies.

As you read through the story, encourage the children to follow along by acting out the poses represented by the keywords in bold letters on each page. The list at the end of the story shows the corresponding poses for each bolded keyword. The illustrations also offer cues for moving through the poses.

Have fun, but please be safe. We hope you enjoy your yoga journey!

For further information and other creative resources, please visit us at:

www.kidsyogastories.com

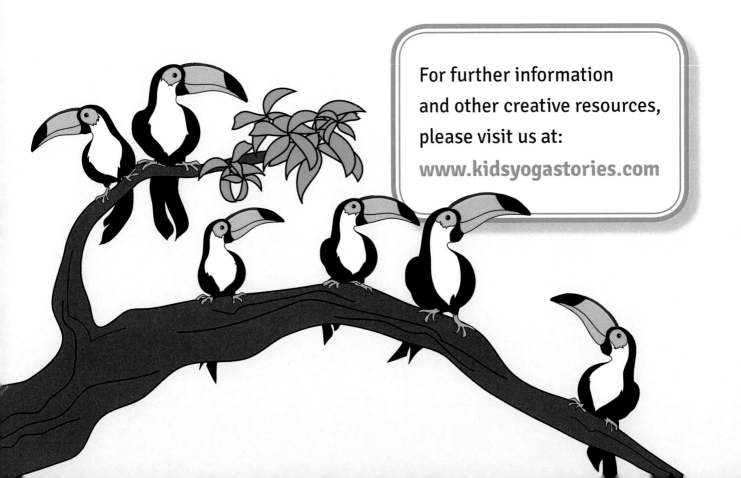

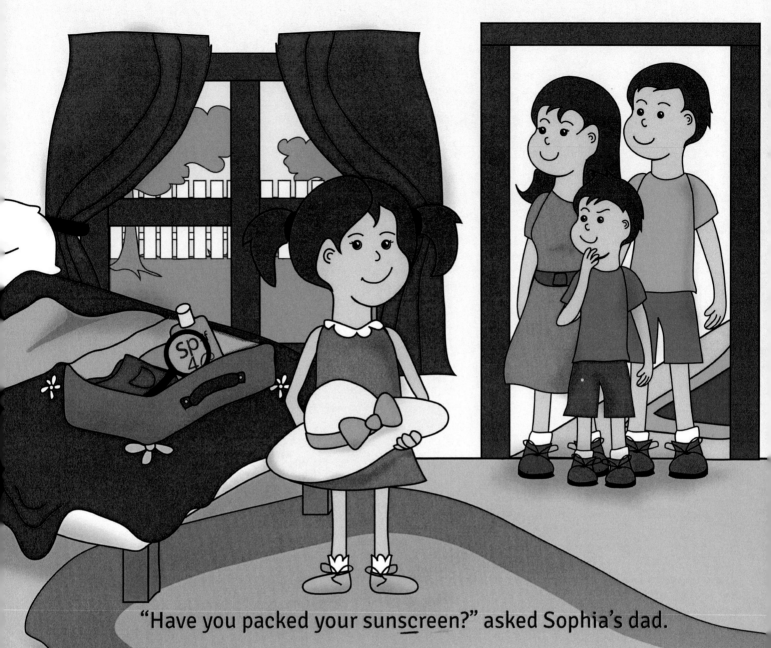

"Have you packed your sunscreen?" asked Sophia's dad.

"Got your sun hat?" asked Sophia's mom.

"And your binoculars and magnifying glass?" asked Sophia's brother, Darren, as he snickered under his breath.

"Yes! Yes! Yes!"

Sophia was almost packed for her family's jungle adventure. Sophia had won the National Nature Writing Contest. Four free tickets to Costa Rica were her prize.

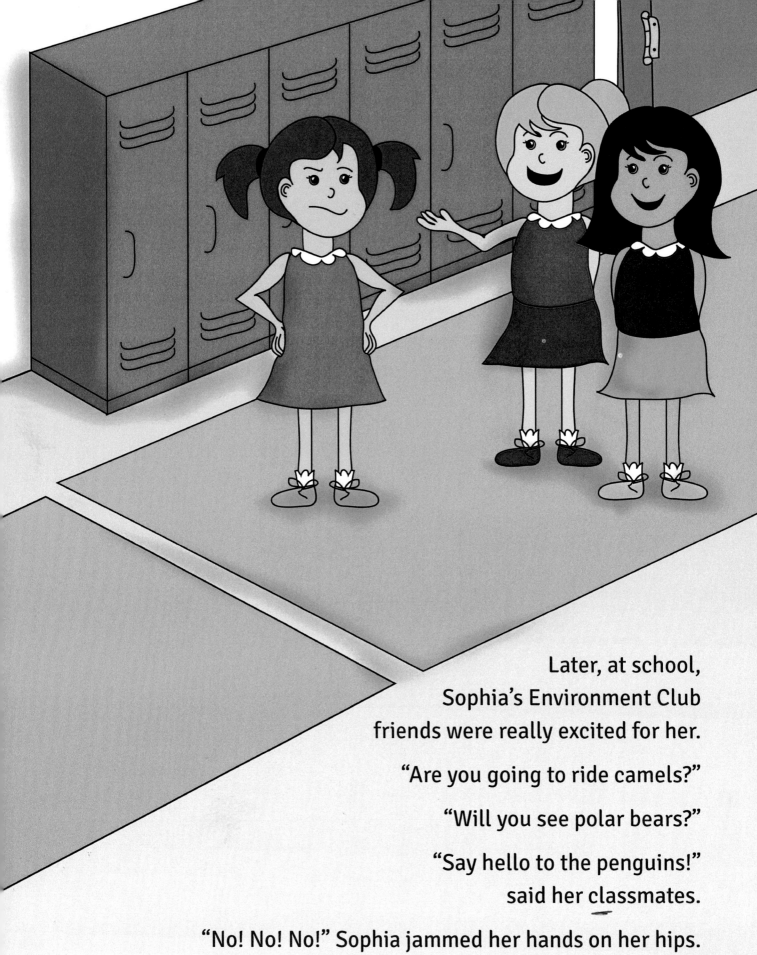

Later, at school,
Sophia's Environment Club
friends were really excited for her.

"Are you going to ride camels?"

"Will you see polar bears?"

"Say hello to the penguins!"
said her classmates.

"No! No! No!" Sophia jammed her hands on her hips.
"Those animals do not live in Costa Rica!"

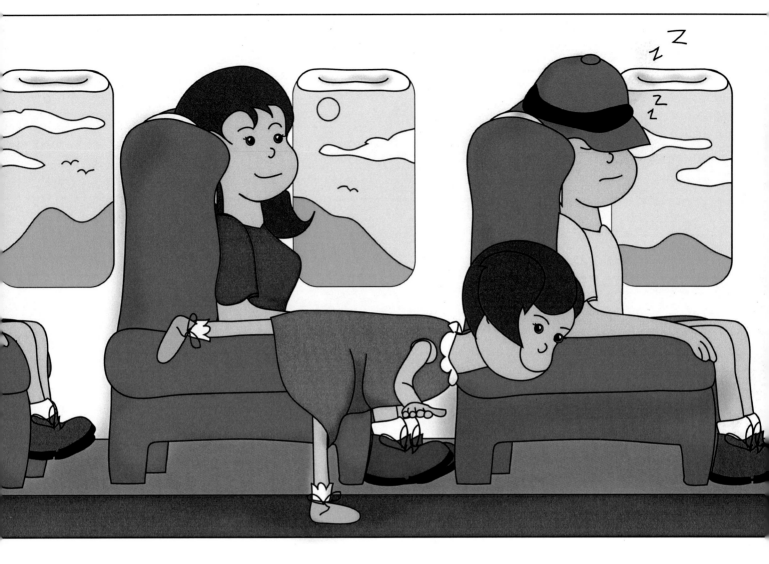

That afternoon, Sophia and her family drove to the airport.

They boarded the **airplane** and flew over tall mountains to Central America.

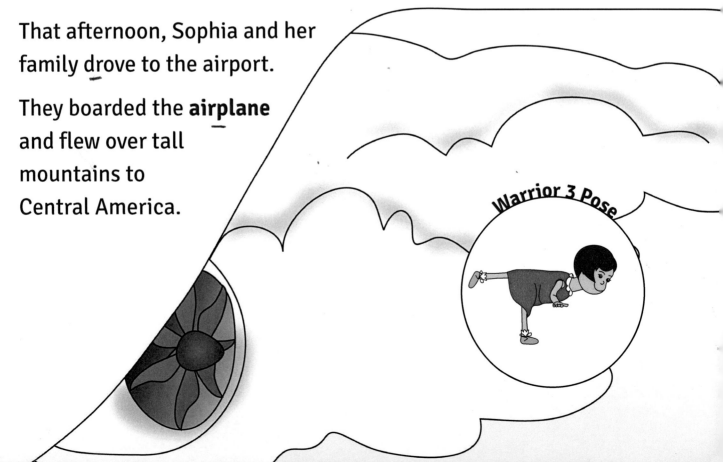

Warrior 3 Pose

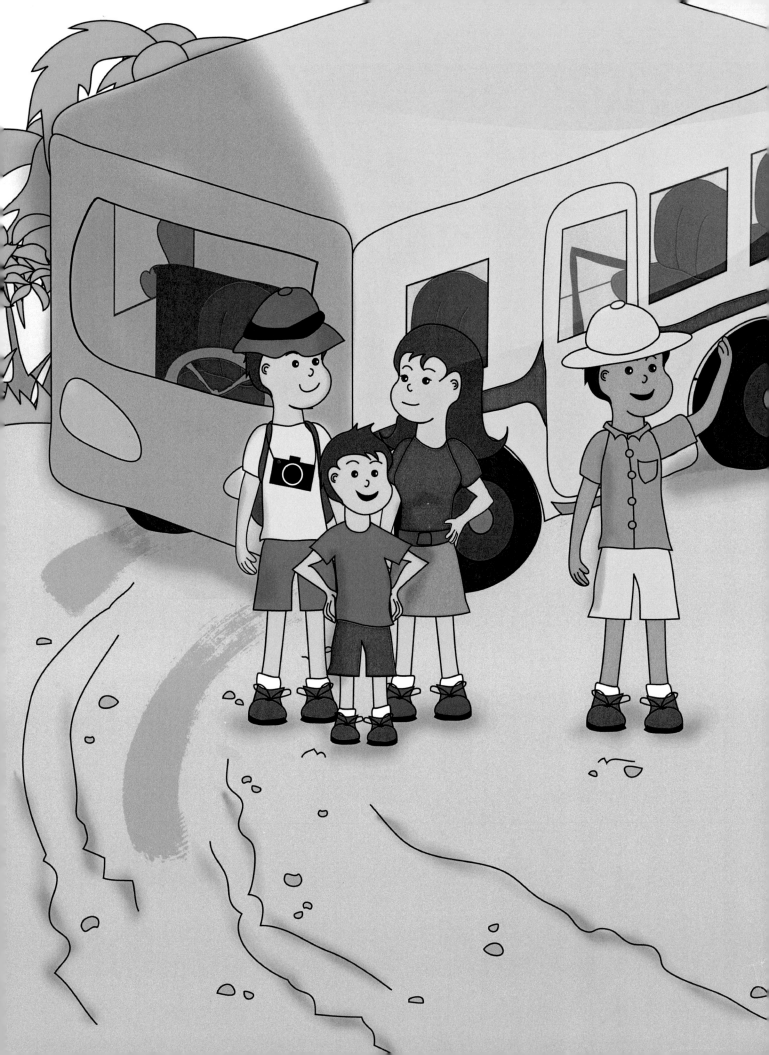

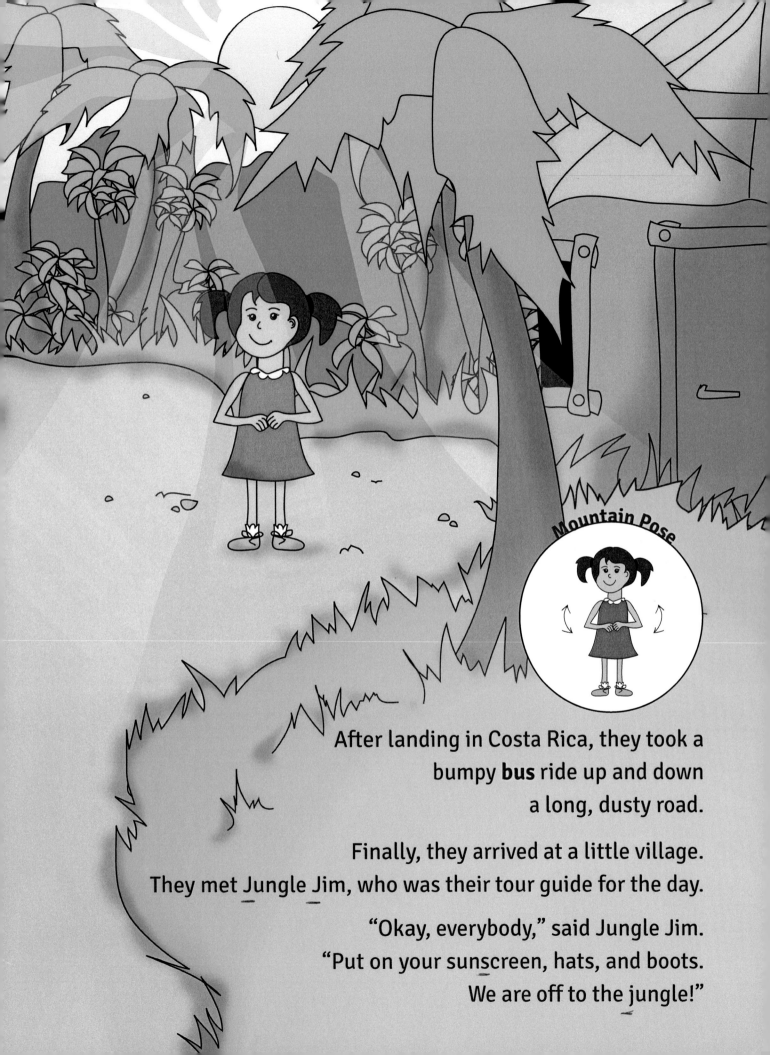

Mountain Pose

After landing in Costa Rica, they took a
bumpy **bus** ride up and down
a long, dusty road.

Finally, they arrived at a little village.
They met Jungle Jim, who was their tour guide for the day.

"Okay, everybody," said Jungle Jim.
"Put on your sunscreen, hats, and boots.
We are off to the jungle!"

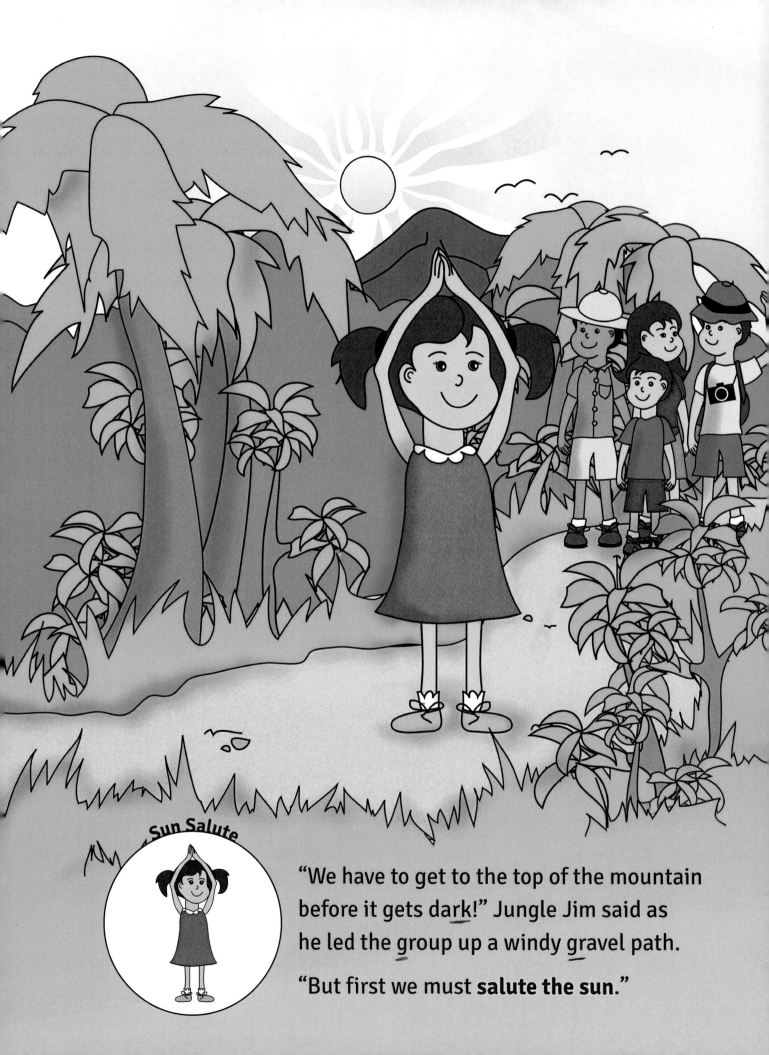

Sun Salute

"We have to get to the top of the mountain before it gets dark!" Jungle Jim said as he led the group up a windy gravel path.

"But first we must **salute the sun.**"

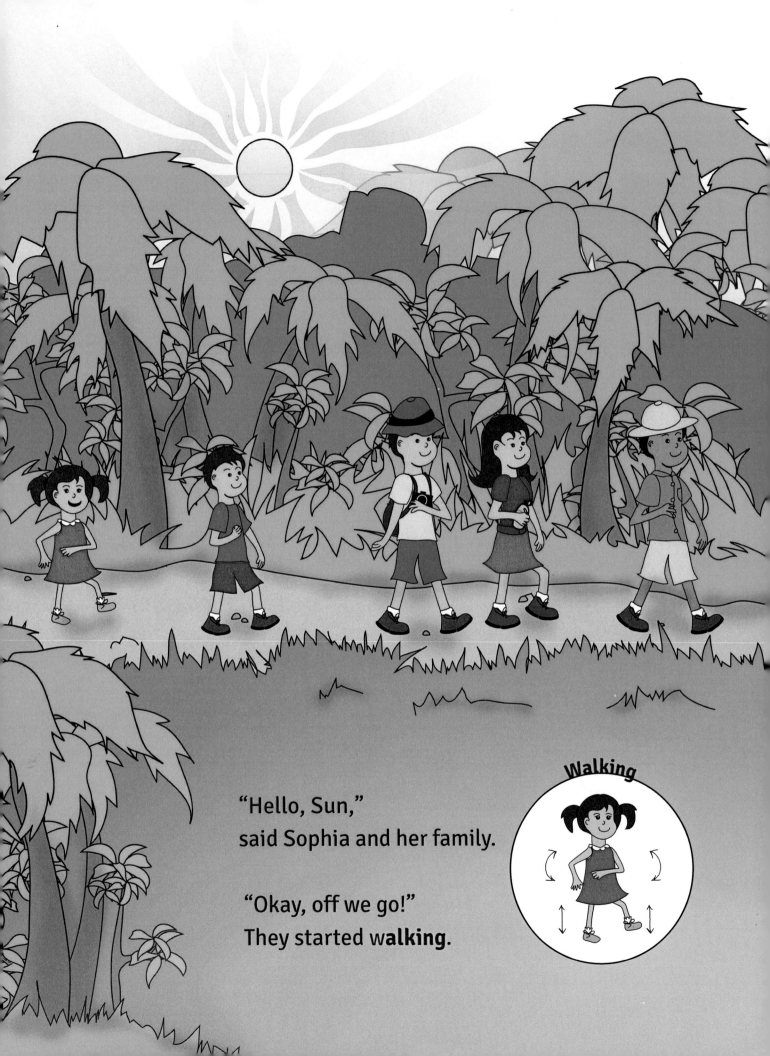

"Hello, Sun,"
said Sophia and her family.

"Okay, off we go!"
They started w**alking**.

Walking

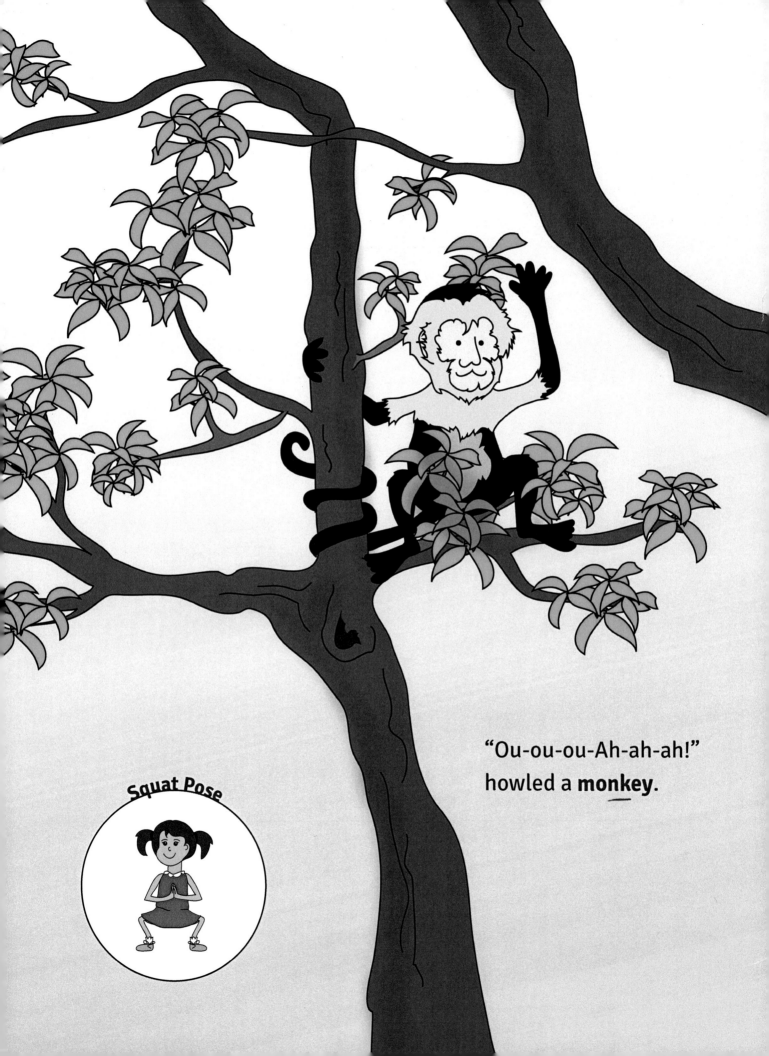

Squat Pose

"Ou-ou-ou-Ah-ah-ah!"
howled a **monkey**.

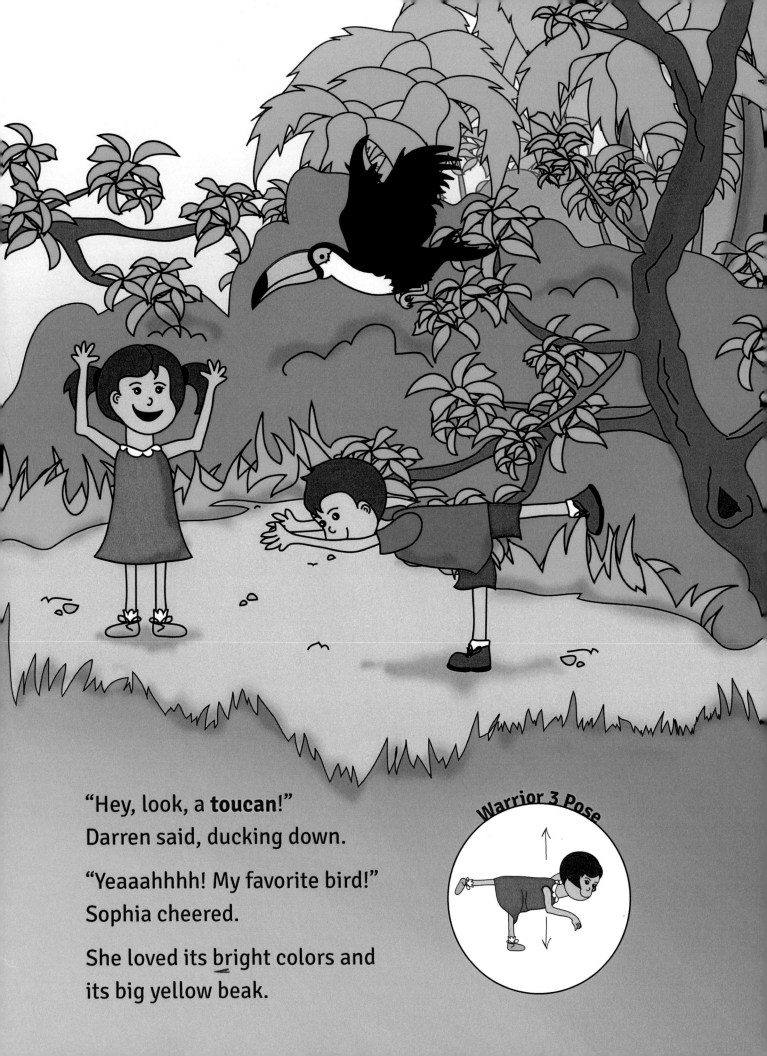

"Hey, look, a **toucan**!"
Darren said, ducking down.

"Yeaaahhhh! My favorite bird!"
Sophia cheered.

She loved its bright colors and
its big yellow beak.

Warrior 3 Pose

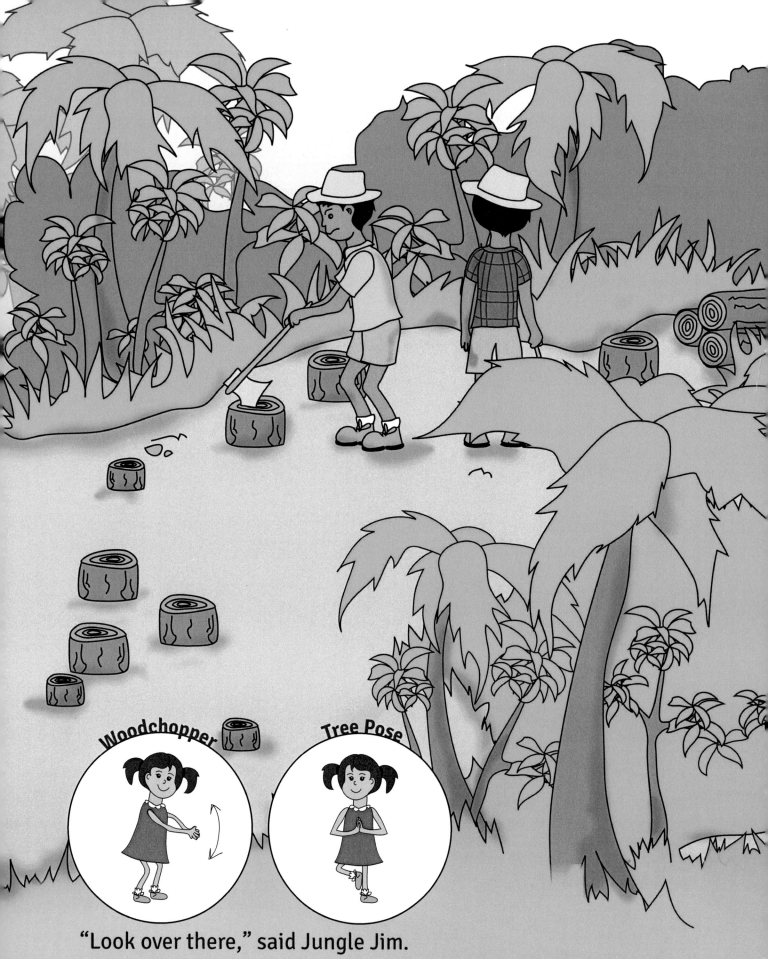

"Look over there," said Jungle Jim.
Woodchoppers are cutting down **trees.**" His face was glum.

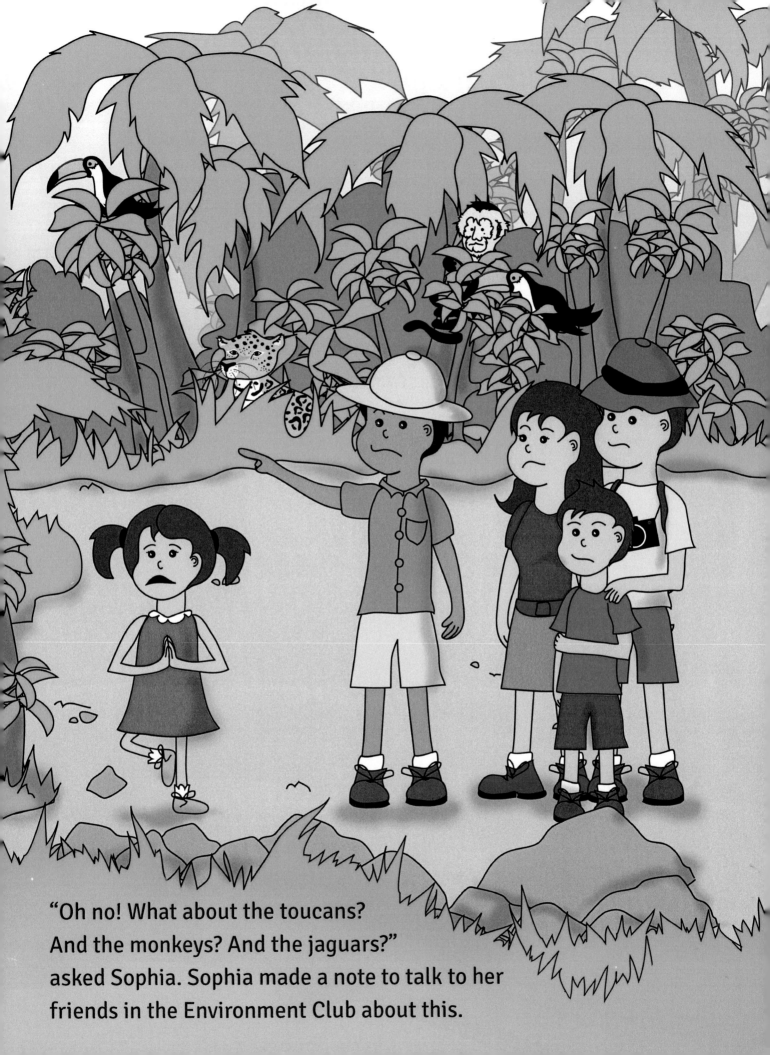

"Oh no! What about the toucans?
And the monkeys? And the jaguars?"
asked Sophia. Sophia made a note to talk to her
friends in the Environment Club about this.

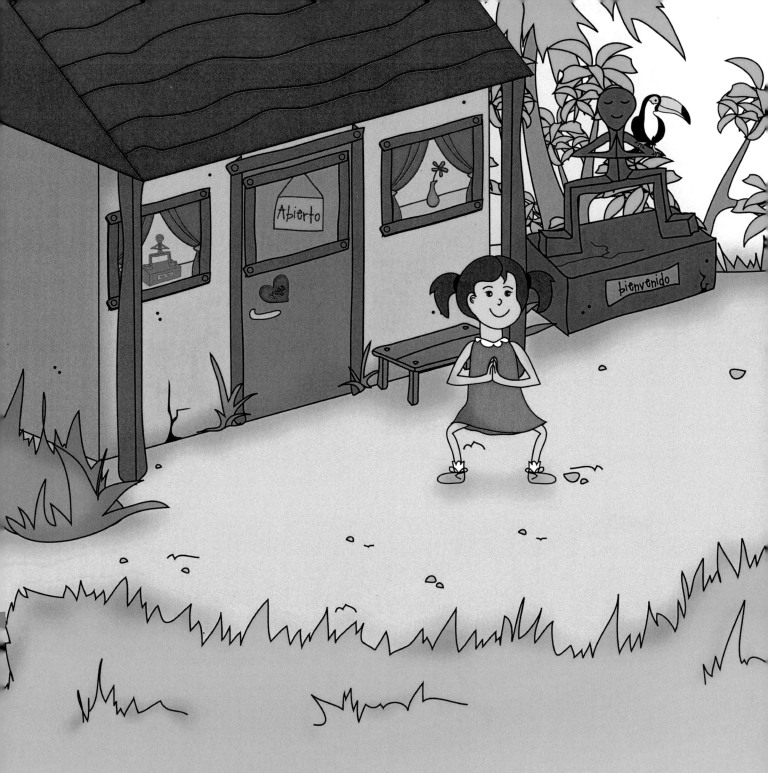

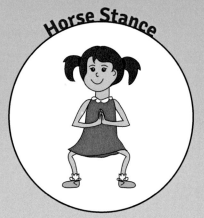

Horse Stance

Jungle Jim and the travelers reached a little store with a **bench** outside.

They stopped to buy some cold drinks.

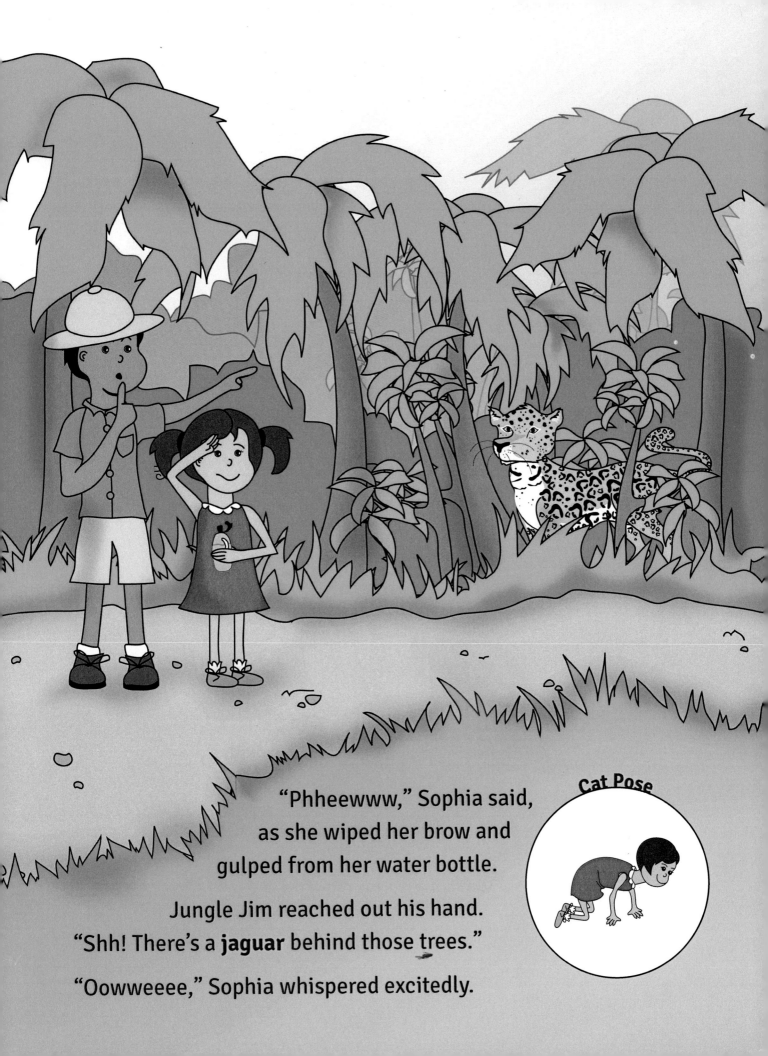

"Phheewww," Sophia said, as she wiped her brow and gulped from her water bottle.

Jungle Jim reached out his hand. "Shh! There's a **jaguar** behind those trees."

"Oowweeee," Sophia whispered excitedly.

Cat Pose

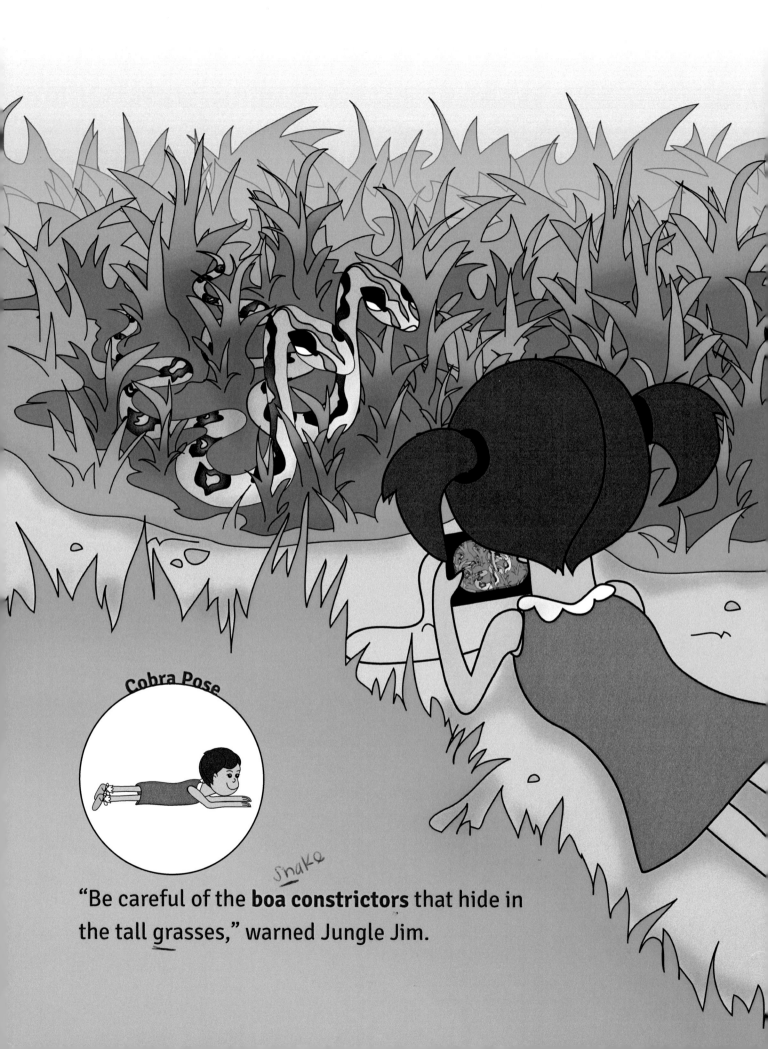

Cobra Pose

snake

"Be careful of the **boa constrictors** that hide in the tall grasses," warned Jungle Jim.

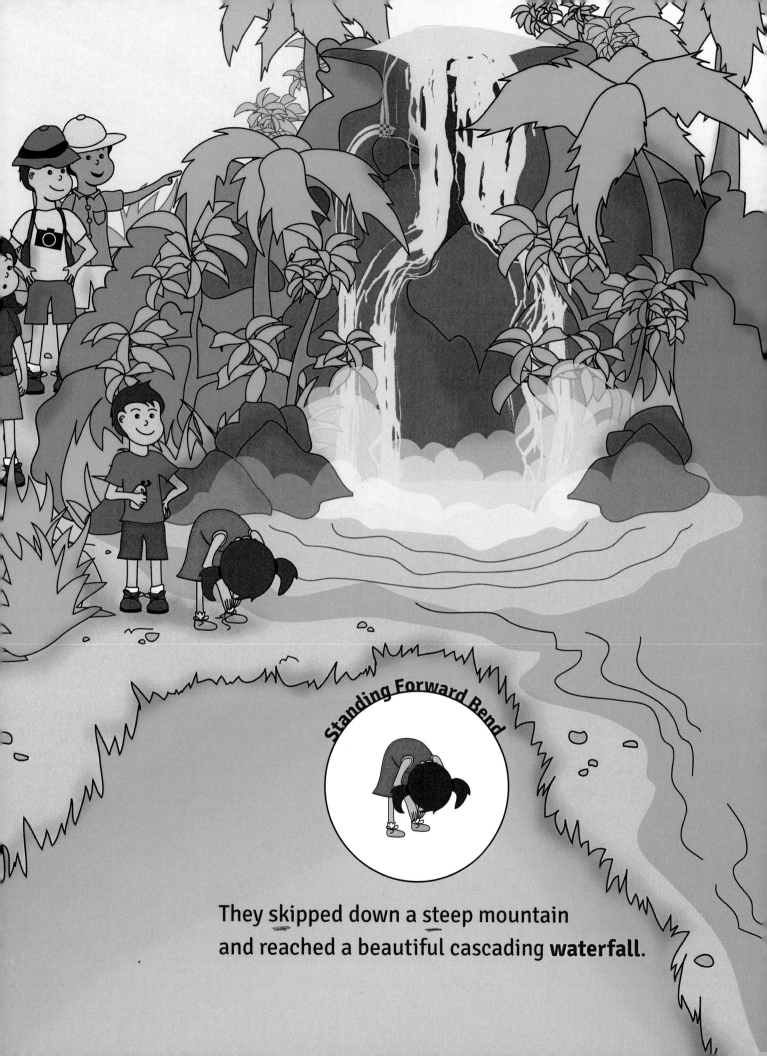

Standing Forward Bend

They skipped down a steep mountain and reached a beautiful cascading **waterfall**.

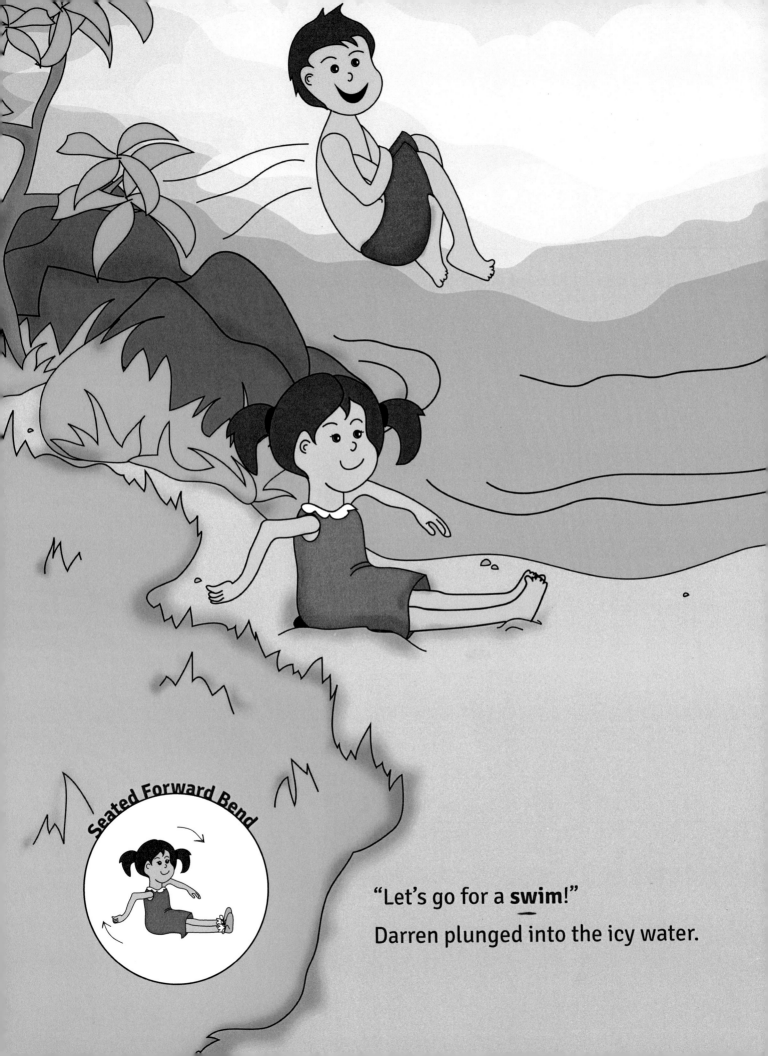

Seated Forward Bend

"Let's go for a **swim**!"
Darren plunged into the icy water.

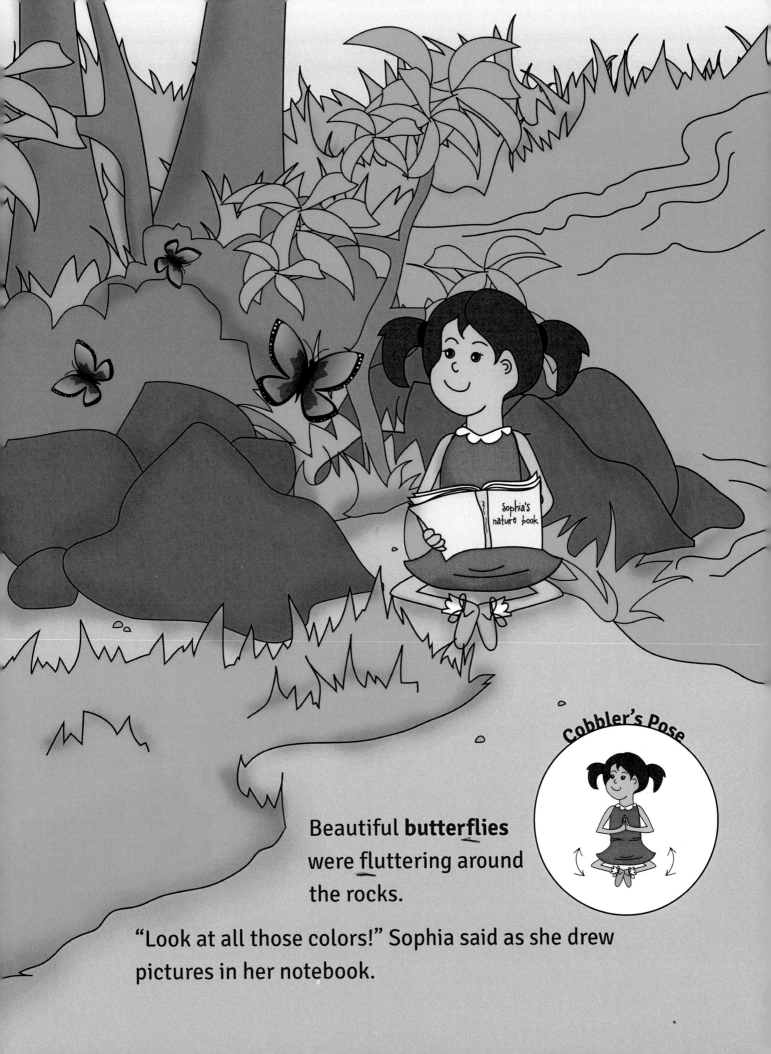

Beautiful **butterflies** were fluttering around the rocks.

"Look at all those colors!" Sophia said as she drew pictures in her notebook.

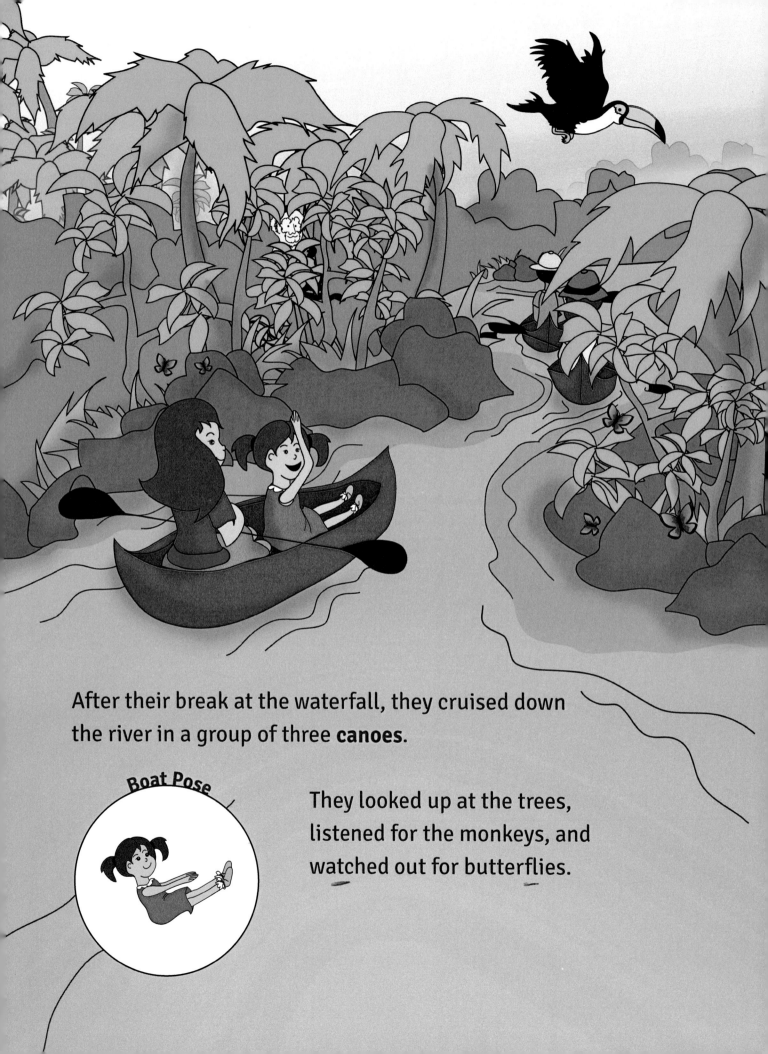

After their break at the waterfall, they cruised down the river in a group of three **canoes**.

Boat Pose

They looked up at the trees, listened for the monkeys, and watched out for butterflies.

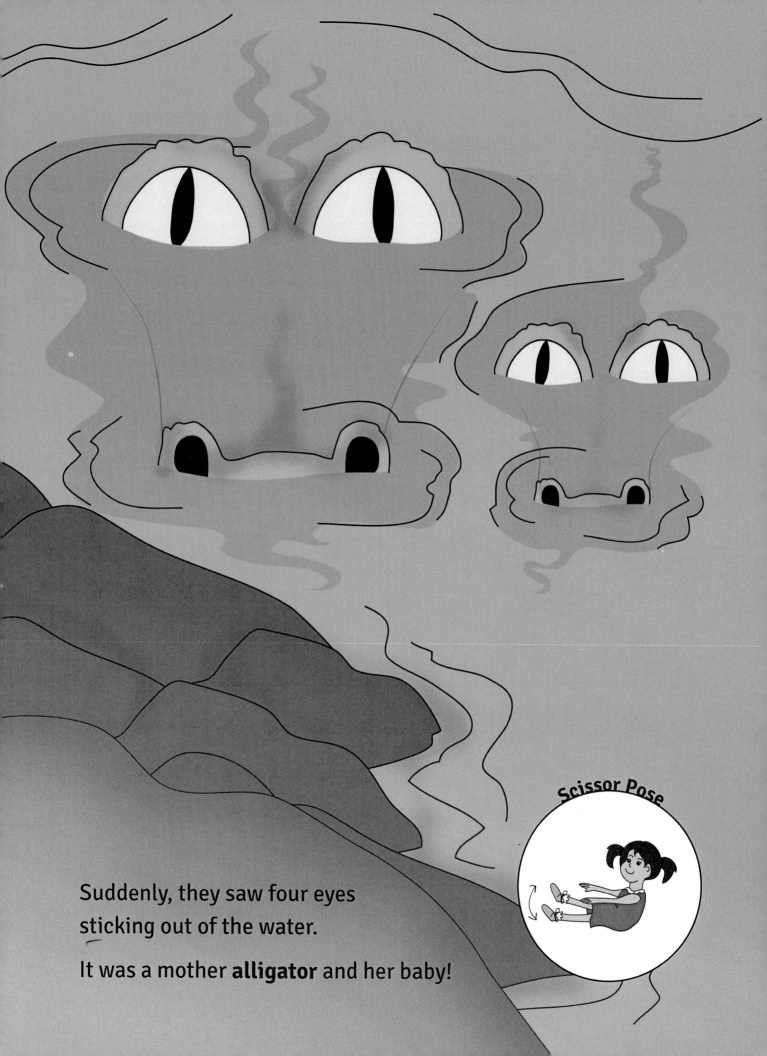

Scissor Pose

Suddenly, they saw four eyes
sticking out of the water.

It was a mother **alligator** and her baby!

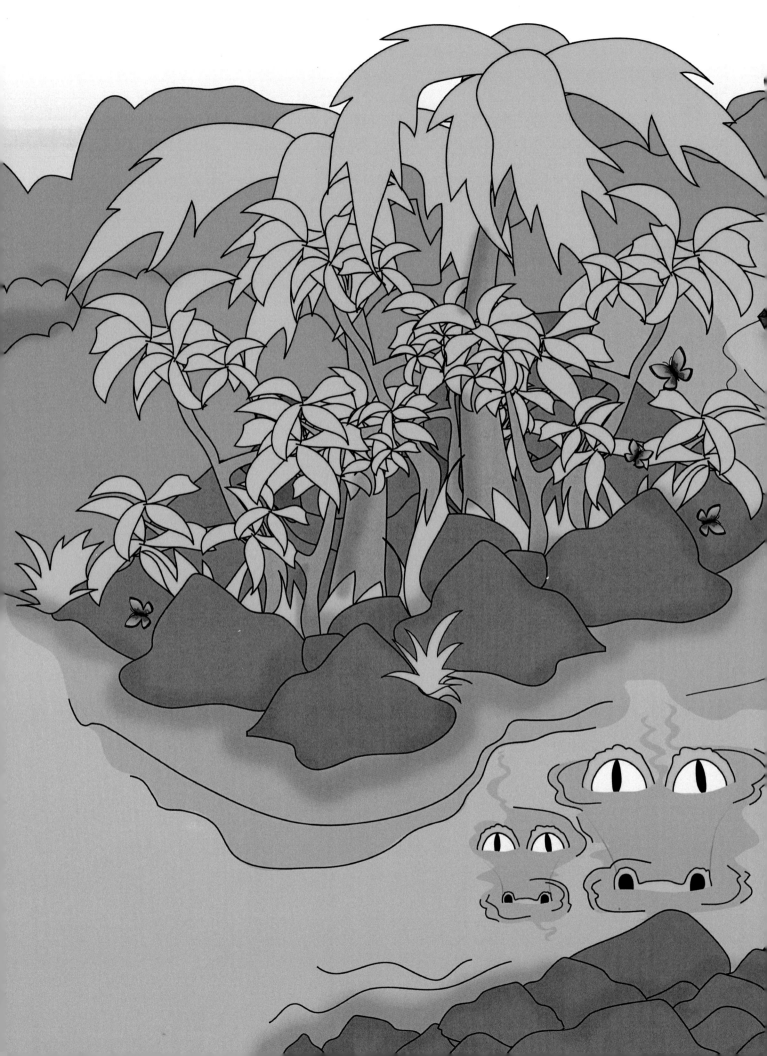

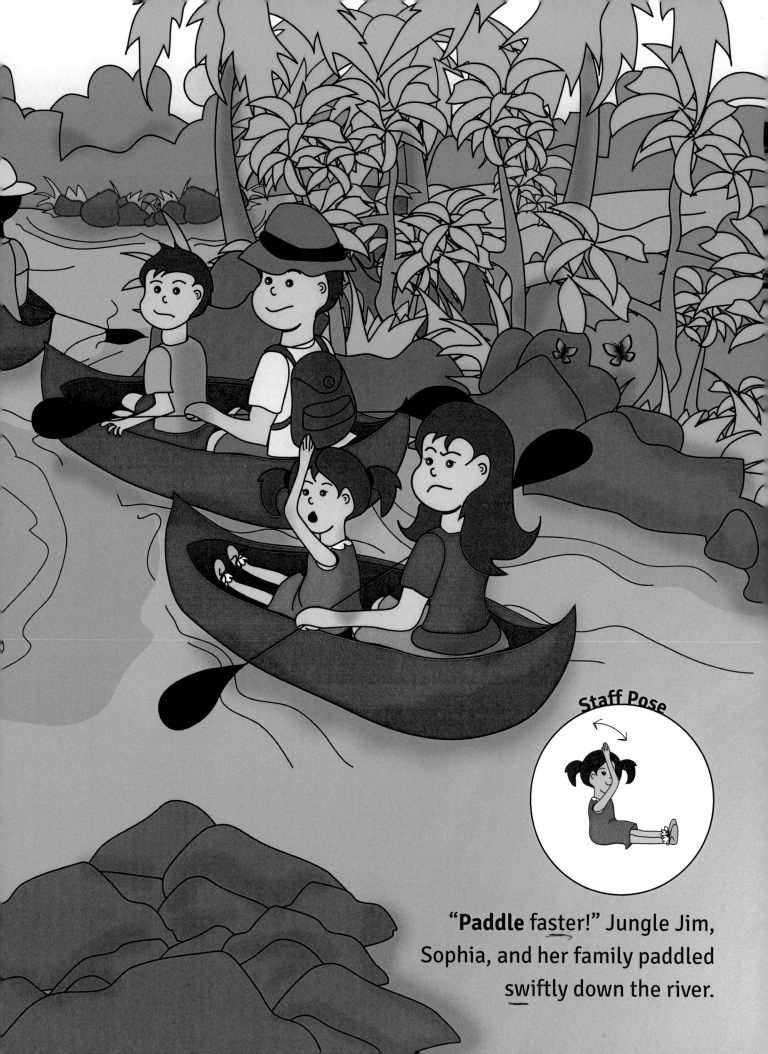

Staff Pose

"**Paddle** faster!" Jungle Jim,
Sophia, and her family paddled
swiftly down the river.

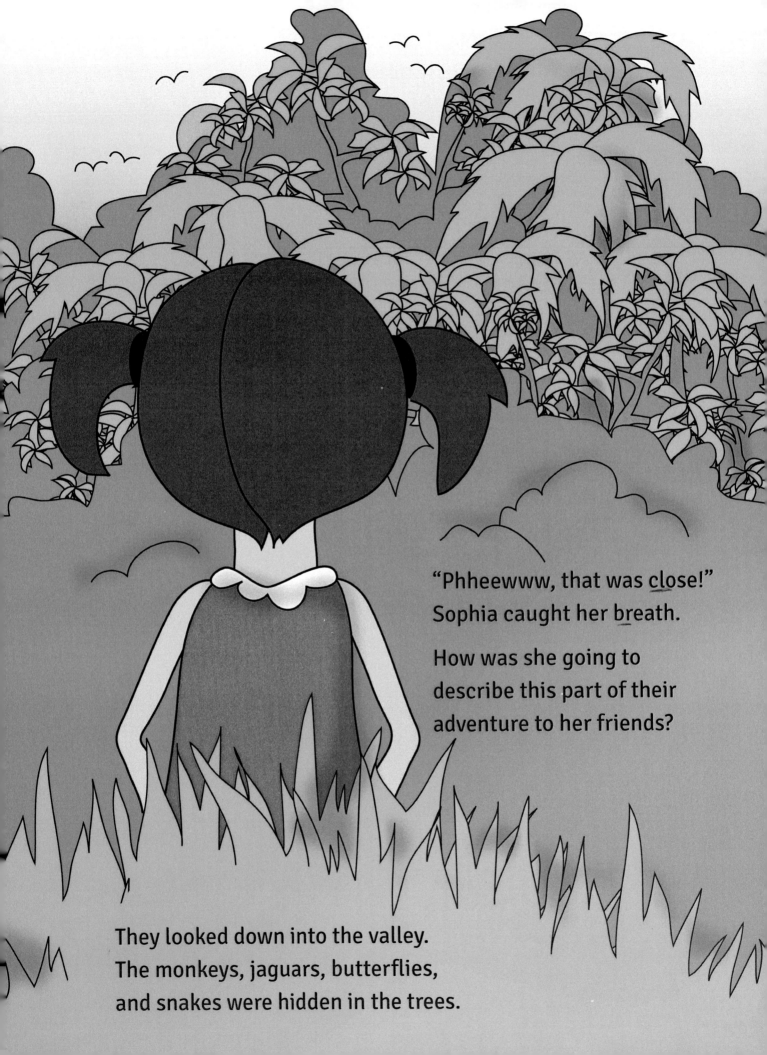

"Phheewww, that was close!"
Sophia caught her breath.

How was she going to
describe this part of their
adventure to her friends?

They looked down into the valley.
The monkeys, jaguars, butterflies,
and snakes were hidden in the trees.

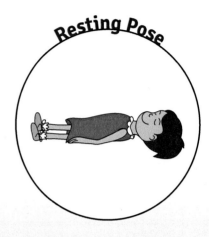

Resting Pose

"Aahhhhhhhh, we made it!"
They were tired but happy.

"Now lie on your back, **relax,** and watch
the stars brighten," said Jungle Jim.

Sophia slowly placed her notebook on her belly
and gently closed her eyes. She wondered where
they would go for their next adventure.

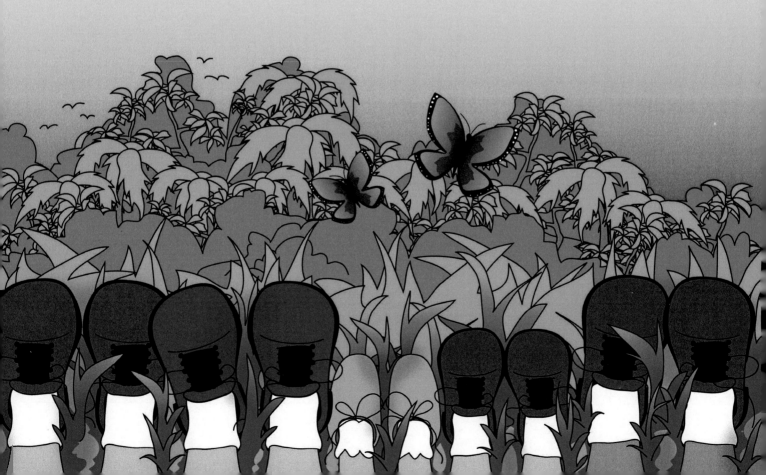

List of Kids Yoga Poses

The following list is intended as a guide only. Please encourage the children's creativity while ensuring their safety.

KEYWORDS	YOGA POSES	DEMONSTRATION
1. Airplane	Warrior 3 Pose	
2. Bus	Mountain Pose	
3. Salute the Sun	Sun Salute	
4. Walking	Walking	
5. Monkey	Squat Pose	
6. Toucan	Warrior 3 Pose	

KEYWORDS	YOGA POSES	DEMONSTRATION
7. Woodchopper	Woodchopper Pose	
8. Trees	Tree Pose	
9. Bench	Horse Stance	
10. Jaguar	Cat Pose	
11. Boa Constrictor	Cobra Pose	
12. Waterfall	Standing Forward Bend	

KEYWORDS	YOGA POSES	DEMONSTRATION
13. Swim	Seated Forward Bend	
14. Butterflies	Cobbler's Pose	
15. Canoes	Boat Pose	
16. Alligator	Scissor Legs	
17. Paddle	Staff Pose	
18. Relax	Resting Pose	

Kids Yoga Stories Guide

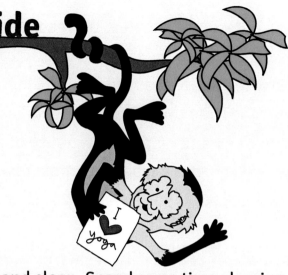

> This guide is intended for kids yoga teachers, primary school teachers, early childhood educators, parents, caregivers, or grandparents — anyone who would like to experience the joy of yoga with young children.

Safety first. Ensure that the space is clear and clean. Spend some time clearing any dangerous objects or unnecessary items. A suitable space could be a spare room in your house, a yoga studio, a classroom, or outside in a park. Wear comfortable clothing and practice barefoot. Wait one to two hours after eating before practicing yoga.

Awaken their senses. Play music that complements your jungle journey. Feel free to add props or pictures to reflect a jungle scene. Or bring in something they can taste to get them in the mood. Make the space inviting and stimulating.

Props are welcome. Lay out a yoga mat for each child in the pattern that works for the space. Mats arranged in a circle seem to work best for younger age groups. Make sure that every child can see you. Towels could also be used instead of yoga mats on a non-slip surface.

Set expectations. At the beginning of the class, review the expectations and guidelines for the session. Be consistent and clear in your communication.

Keep it real and meaningful. Capture their imagination and link the topic back to their lives.

Be enthusiastic. Children will feed off your enthusiasm. Tell them stories of your own that are related to the book's topic. They will be more engaged if they can see that you are enjoying yourself.

Sequence your journey. We recommend that you follow the sequence of the yoga poses described in the story, because they have been specifically sequenced to create a well-balanced and safe kids yoga class. Feel free to add more poses, but try to keep the poses closely linked to the sequence. For example, if you are doing the standing poses sequence of story, feel free to add different standing poses. Avoid dropping down into a forward bend during the standing poses sequence, but instead wait until the story takes you down to similar poses.

Repetition is effective. Feel free to repeat the story as many times as the children are engaged. Ask the children to say or predict the next pose in the journey.

"Ou-ou-ou-Ah-ah-ah!"

Lighten up and have fun. A children's yoga class is not as formal as an adult class. Allow the children time to explore the postures and movements. Focus on the journey and avoid teaching perfectly aligned poses. The journey is intended to be joyful and fun.

Explain the intention and purpose. Explain to your young "travelers" where your pretend journey will take them and how the session will unfold. We recommend reading the story together first and then moving through the poses during the second reading. Do what suits you.

Cater to the age group. Use the **Kids Yoga Stories** as a guide, but make adaptations according to the age group of the children in your class. Feel free to lengthen or shorten the story to ensure that the children are fully engaged throughout your time together. Our recommendation is to work with children ages four to eight, as they are able to concentrate for longer periods of time, enjoy playful movement, and love storytelling. Break the journey down into a couple of poses for each session if you're working with ages three to five. Add more poses and extend the ideas if you're working with children over six years old. They might write their own stories, invent their own poses, read the stories on their own, read books about the topic, take pictures of themselves in the poses, or paint pictures of the poses and animals.

Be mindful of the children's abilities. Focus on the strengths of the children. Be aware of any physical or mental challenges that the children, or a single child, are bringing to the session.

Adapt to the group size. We recommend a group size of about eight to ten children, but you could do these stories with one to thirty children. We also recommend a class length of about thirty minutes to one hour. For groups of ten or more, it would be a good idea to read the story first as a group, discuss the poses, talk about your expectations, and then read the story again while moving through the poses.

Foster compassion and kindness. Model and guide an experience where compassion and kindness are integral. Teach the children to follow this motto: "Respect Yourself, Respect Others, Respect Property, and Respect the Environment."

Be open and accepting. Encourage the strengths of each child and allow them to experience feelings of success and acceptance.

Ooze creativity, imagination, and abundance. Encourage each child to tap into their own creativity and imagination through movement and breath. Welcome quiet times for reflection. Pause lots. Remember, it's not the end result, but the journey where miracles happen...

About Kids Yoga Stories

We hope that you enjoyed your **Kids Yoga Stories** experience.

Visit our website, www.kidsyogastories.com, to:

Receive updates. For updates, contest giveaways, articles, and activity ideas, sign up for our **Kids Yoga Stories Newsletter.**

Connect with us. Please share with us about your yoga journey. Send us pictures of yourself practicing the poses or reading the story. Describe your journey on our social media pages (Facebook, Pinterest, Google+, or Twitter).

Check out free stuff. Read our articles on books, yoga, parenting, and travel. Download one of our kids yoga lesson plans or coloring pages.

Read or write a review. Read what others have to say about our books or post your own review on Amazon or on our website. We'd love to hear how you enjoyed **Sophia's Jungle Adventure.**

Thank you for your support in spreading our message of integrating learning, movement and fun.

Giselle
Kids Yoga Stories

www.kidsyogastories.com
info@kidsyogastories.com
www.facebook.com/kidsyogastories
www.pinterest.com/kidsyogastories
www.twitter.com/kidsyogastories
www.amazon.com/author/giselleshardlow

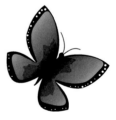

About the Author

Giselle Shardlow draws from her experiences as a teacher, traveler, mother, and yogi to write her yoga stories for kids. The purpose of her yoga books is to foster happy, healthy, and globally educated children. She lives in Boston with her husband and daughter.

About the Illustrator

Emily Gedzyk is a world traveler who draws her artistic inspiration from the places she's visited and the people in her life. She hopes to continue her journeys to new, exciting places and to teach everyone she meets that it's never too early or too late to go out into the world on their own adventures.

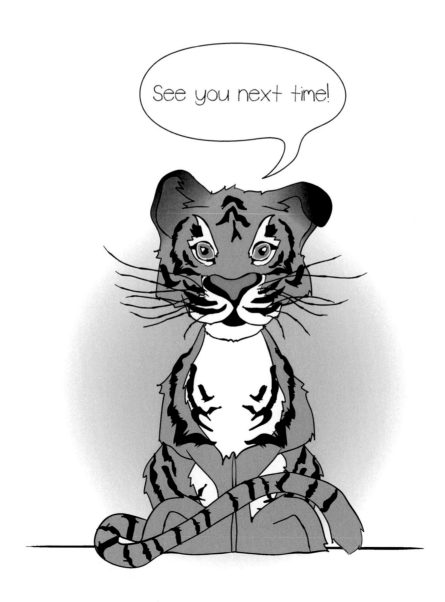

Other Yoga Stories by Giselle Shardlow

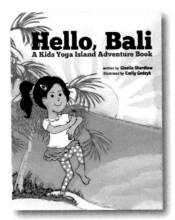

Hello, Bali

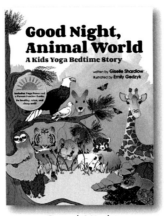

Good Night, Animal World

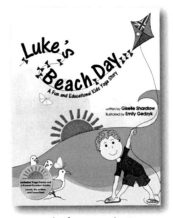

Luke's Beach Day

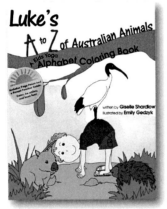

Luke's A to Z of Australian Animals Coloring Book

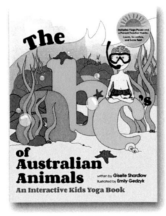

The ABC's of Australian Animals

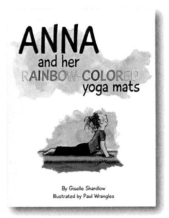

Anna and her Rainbow-Colored Yoga Mats

Many of the books above are available in Spanish and eBook format.

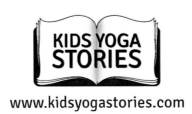

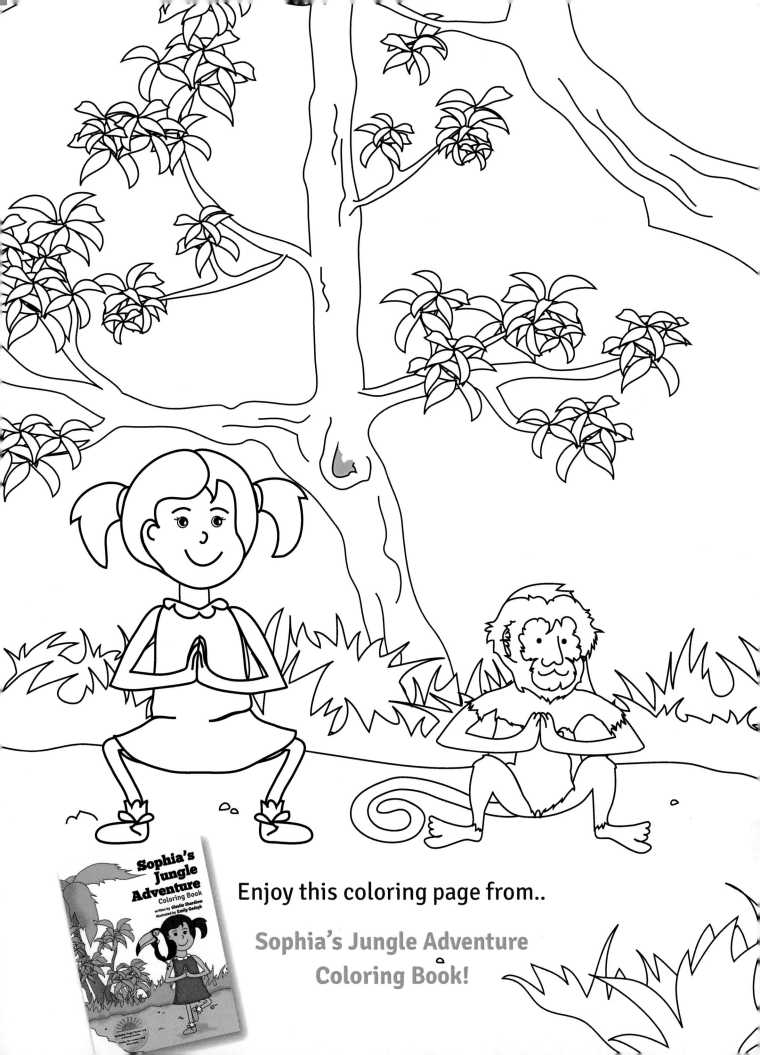

Enjoy this coloring page from..

Sophia's Jungle Adventure
Coloring Book!

Made in the USA
Middletown, DE
07 July 2016